For My Sweet, Sweet

Christina

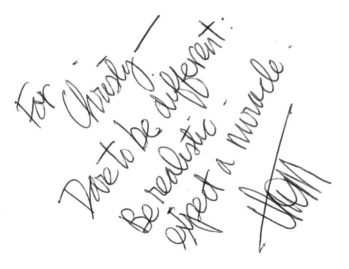

For Christy —
Dare to be different.
Be realistic.
Expect a miracle

"I'm thin but fun."

-- Woody Allen

THE COMMON SENSE APPROACH

TO

A

HEALTHY LIFESTYLE

Thom Slagle

Illustrated
by

Beth W. Reasoner

PWP/Pacific Word Publishing, Palo Alto, California

THE COMMON SENSE APPROACH

TO

A

HEALTHY LIFESTYLE

Published by:

Pacific Word Publishing
4250 Terman Drive, Suite 104
Palo Alto, CA 94306

First Printing 1993
Printed in the United States of America

Publisher's Cataloging in Publication Data
Slagle, Thom
The Common Sense Approach to a Healthy Lifestyle
1. Health   I. Title
2. Fitness
3. Diet
4. Self-Improvement

Library of Congress Catalog Card Number: 93-84106

ISBN: 0-9636421-7-0: 15.95 Softcover

TABLE OF CONTENTS

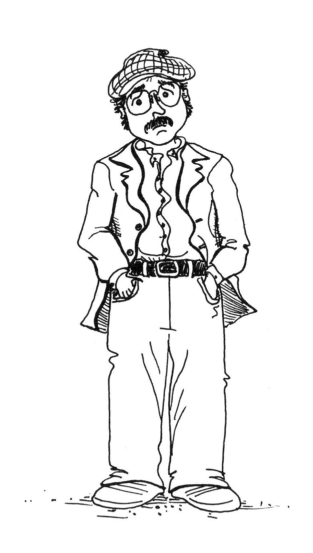

ABOUT THE AUTHOR

Dr. Herman Hepner never had any doubts about his career choice, following his mother, father, grandfather, and two uncles into the field of medicine. For thirty-seven years, he was a dedicated physician in the same small midwestern community that welcomed him in 1953. Dr. Hepner was well-known for his gentle bedside manner and compassion in his approach to medicine. He passed away in November of 1992 from cancer of the bone marrow, from which he had suffered for 1 1/2 years. Dr. Hepner is remembered by family, friends, and colleagues as a quiet, devoted family man.

On the other hand, Thom Slagle never could make up his mind as to what he wanted to be when he finally grew up. So he tried several occupations, none of which really interested or amused him, before settling on life as a writer and book publisher. He has written several short stories, a collection of poetry, and a screenplay, and has several projects in line to be published in the near future. He and his business partner, Christina, have been married for five years and share their Palo Alto, California home with their six sons.

PREFACE

The Common Sense Approach to a Healthy Lifestyle is *not* a diet program. Diets require the participant to *give up* certain great tasting foods and, on top of that, they *insist upon* the dieter getting up and exercising to make the program work. Besides, I've always suspected that virtually all diets were created by skinny guys in white lab coats who really didn't have a clue as to the inherent problems that we People of Excessive Weight must constantly confront.

That's why the *Common Sense Approach* was created. It *was not* developed by one of these montrous skinny geek-like creatures. No, the *Approach* was created by a fat person who was -- excuse the pun -- *fed up* with being fat and out of shape, and thoroughly frustrated by his inability to lose weight by conventional means. With the help of his trusted family physician, the *Common Sense Approach* was methodically sketched out through a process of trial-and-error as various obstacles and hurdles had to be dealt with. When something didn't work, it was analyzed and dissected to find out *why*, and then the adjustments were made in the program to compensate for it. And it worked like a charm. How do I know? **I was that fat person**.

The *Common Sense Approach* will teach you how to develop that ever-elusive concept called ***willpower***. And, you'll find the *Approach* easy to follow. **You won't have to sacrifice** a single, solitary food **to enjoy the benefits**! To the contrary, **the *Approach* actually *encourages* you to eat those things you love.**

By the way, as you'll discover upon reading this book, I love to eat and hate to exercise primarily because I'm lazy and very anti-diet. Food for thought. *Bon Appetit*!

ACKNOWLEDGEMENTS

The author wishes to acknowledge the invaluable assistance of Beth W. Reasoner, whose illustrations give life to ordinary and mere words, and whose friendship has been stalwart and unwavering through the good times and bad; Julia Robinson, PhD, for her endorsement of, and support for, the behavioral techniques employed in the *Approach*; and, to Marian Hepner, without whose blessings and consent this book would not have been possible.

But mostly, the author would like to acknowledge the late Herman Hepner, MD, whose wisdom and inspiration led directly to the creation of the *Common Sense Approach to a Healthy Lifestyle*. Without his influence and guidance, this book could not have been written.

And finally, to the countless others who directly or indirectly influenced, encouraged, and otherwise championed my endeavors to win the Battle of the Bulge, I extend my heartfelt gratitude.

WARNING -- DISCLAIMER

This book is designed to provide an agenda for, and insight into, losing weight. It is sold with the understanding that the publisher and the author are not engaged in rendering medical or other professional health services. As with any program involved with health, fitness, and weight loss, it is incumbent upon each individual participant to seek the advice of a trusted physician or other healthcare professional prior to pursuing any planned agenda, including this one.

Every effort has been made to make this book as complete and accurate as possible. However, there may be mistakes both typographical and in content. Therefore, this text should be used only as a general guide and not as the ultimate source of health/fitness information.

The purpose of this book is to educate and entertain, and to share the experiences of the author in his efforts to modify his lifestyle. The author and Pacific Word Publishing shall have neither liability nor responsibility to any person or entity with respect to any loss or damage caused or alleged to be caused directly or indirectly by the information contained in this book.

WARNING -- DISCLAIMER

IN MEMORIAM

HERMAN H. HEPNER, MD

(1927 - 1992)

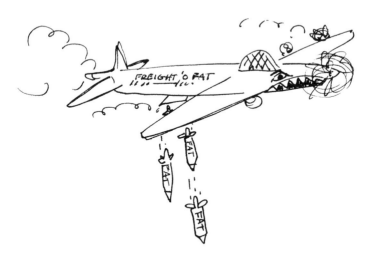

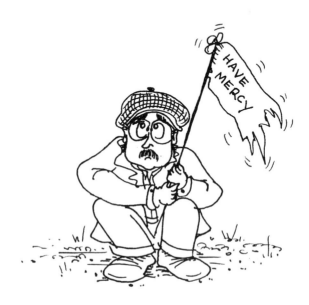

CHAPTER ONE
The Winds of War

This is a personal account of my struggle to lose weight and change my lifestyle. After years of submitting to a variety of diets, health plans, and ritualistic hogwash, I was convinced that I was destined to remain for life a Person of Excessive Weight. Not that I wanted to be, or that my body -- other than my stomach -- really resembled the stereotypical picture of obesity but, quite honestly, I loved to eat and hated to exercise -- an extremely dangerous combination -- and these programs, while suggesting they could make me lean and healthy, forced me to cut out foods that I loved and cherished, and demanded that I establish a regimen of rigorous exercise in order for them to make me thin. Nice try.

I think I tried to follow every diet plan that was published from the late 60s on; the longest I could actually endure any of them without cheating was maybe three days. Why? Because I lacked the *willpower* to stay away from the foods that I loved, and I lacked the initiative and drive to get out and exercise -- even though the plans promised me a better life and a nice, toned body in exchange. Nonsense. I was fat and lazy, and easily discouraged by all the work involved with losing weight.

Then in late 1970, certain unforeseeable events happened that changed my attitude about how I wanted to live and, consequently, altered my lifestyle. Those events breathed life into a program of smart eating and a healthier lifestyle -- without sacrifice -- that has proven successful for me, a naturally lazy, lethargic guy who was prone to being overweight but not necessarily liking it.

I call the program the *Common Sense Approach to a Healthy Lifestyle* because it is predicated on just that: common sense. The only alleged expert I consulted was my family physician, mostly as a matter of prudence rather than to seek advice although, in retrospect, his wisdom and approach in dealing with me were incredibly influential and inspirational -- and directly responsible for my ultimate success in losing weight. In developing the *Approach*, I analyzed the reasons why I could not be true to other programs created by so-called experts and then made allowances for them. I designed it to reduce my excess weight *gradually*, the theory being that not only is it healthier to lose weight a little at a time, but it is more inclined to stay off if lost in this manner. It was a matter of trial and error -- common sense, again -- with few adjustments and no concessions to speak of.

What began as merely a self-designed *personal* weight loss program ultimately became a new lifestyle even though I hadn't planned it that way. Fact of the matter is: the *Common Sense Approach to a Healthy Lifestyle* was developed by a person who has continuously waged a battle of the bulge -- not by people who profess to know what is best for people like you and me. And, by golly, the *Approach* worked for me, and has been successful for over two decades. Okay, there was one slight relapse, but I beat that too. Hey, isn't that what years of research is all about anyway?

Obviously, I cannot guarantee that you will succeed in losing weight on my plan; but I do know that if you read this book and visualize the concepts of the *Common Sense*

Approach, you will have to agree that *it could actually work* for you. Because it makes sense -- common sense.

So, let's get with it. There's a war to be fought that we will finally win -- the Battle of the Bulge!

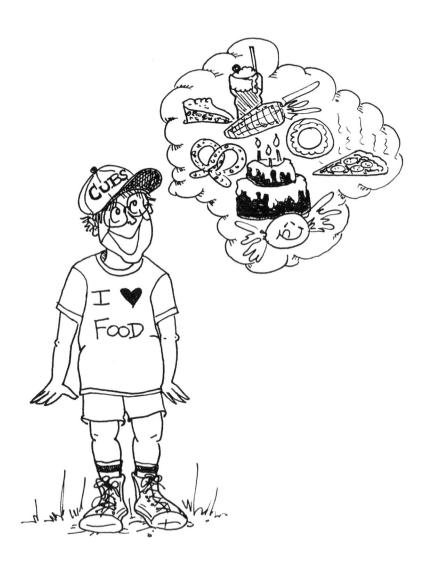

CHAPTER TWO
A Call to Arms

It's certainly no fun being fat. I speak from experience: I was the proverbial fat kid in the neighborhood, the one whose t-shirt was always so tight that the ridges of fat stuck out around my waist like some sort of relief map of the Rocky Mountains. From my pre-teen years through my days as a teenager, the weight hung around my middle announcing to the world that I was unfit and miserable; a sorry slob whose life-skills were pretty much dysfunctional. In other words, *I was a pig.*

For as long as I can remember, whenever sides were being chosen for games of sport or recreation, I was almost always the last person picked from the group of kids along the sidelines. It didn't matter that I was as good as, or better than, most of the others selected before me; what counted to my classmates and friends was that I was overweight and that meant -- automatically -- that everybody else *had* to be better. I couldn't run as fast, nor maneuver as well; I couldn't shoot the basketball with as much accuracy, nor hit a baseball as far. In the minds of my playmates and peers, I was fat and just plain no good. Period.

No matter the taunting jeers of my classmates and the looks of disdain from complete strangers -- slender people mostly, I might add -- I was pretty much a happy kid. A cheerful disposition and disarming wit shielded me from the sting of criticism and was, despite my weight problem, a magnet in attracting more than my share of acquaintances and friends. My life was basically pretty serene and enjoyable. I just had a couple of minor problems: I loved to eat and hated to exercise. It didn't make me a bad person, mind you, despite what others would try to get me to believe with their relentless taunts. Actually, my life nowhere resembled a shambles.

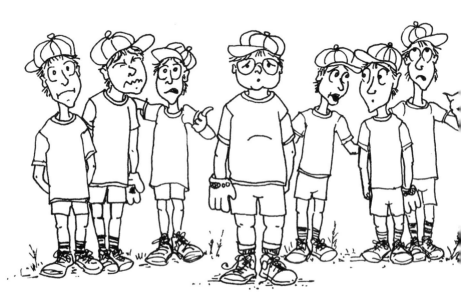

My love of eating was not the result of some deeply-rooted psychological trauma that reared its ugly head and manifested itself in my need to devour the rest of the half-eaten chocolate layer cake or to help myself to seconds, thirds, and sometimes, fourths of the nightly dinners. Fact was, I had a loving, nurturing childhood; I simply had a real weakness for all those wonderfully tantalizing baked goods and great tasting dishes that were being conjured up in the kitchen on a daily basis -- each aroma my personal siren of temptation. So, to hell with all those psychological profiles and studies that report otherwise. What do those guys know *anyway*! Heavy-set people are not bad people anymore than slender, fit people are. My guess is that most of those studies were supervised and analyzed by really skinny people who have this abject prejudice against People of Excessive Weight, and that they simply want to toy and fiddle with our emotional balance by condemning our practice of stuffing ourselves with dishes of delight, and just make us feel like crap. It's a mind-control thing with them. Sort of like a bunch of little latter-day Hitlers trying to throw their weight around. Well, that ain't gonna happen, I'm telling you ...

My problem wasn't complex at all. I had this enormous appetite and I ate all I wanted to satisfy the pangs of hunger that coaxed me from inside my ever-expanding stomach. Simple as that. I avoided virtually all forms of known exercise and ignored the mild protestations of my parents and other relatives, and all my friends concerning my eating habits. I loved to eat and that's that.

So what changed my mind? In late 1970, I was nineteen years old, cocky and arrogant -- and about forty pounds overweight. At least, if you believe those statistical charts that are published by so-called experts (no doubt, thin ones) that profess to know such things. I was still a happy-go-lucky person, quick with a smile and a joke, and still eating damned near twice my weight in food at each sitting. In other words, nothing much had changed to this point in my life. I was eating whatever I wanted whenever I wanted, and exercise to me was having to hoist myself up from my easy chair in front of the television to grab another bag of cookies or make another sandwich. Or both.

The day before Thanksgiving that year an event occurred which would have a profound effect on me and my family. My father, always a picture of strength and health by my way of thinking, suffered a heart attack. While not massive, that fact did not diminish the fear and anxiety that ripped through the veil of contentment behind which my family lived. There is a fine line that separates Life from Death and, for the first time, my family was forced to examine just how fine a line it really was. Up close and personal. And for the first time in my life, I was truly scared. My father was no longer strong and independent; rather, now he was vulnerable and completely dependent on others for life. Quite frankly, it scared the hell out of me. If ever two people were cast from the same mold, it was my father and me. Suddenly, I was staring at the inevitability of Death lying motionless in a hospital bed with tubes and needles and monitors and nurses and doctors everywhere. Sure, it was my father. But the face I saw was mine.

I realized at that moment that, unless I preferred death to life, I was going to have to do something dramatic about my devil-may-care approach to life, and my expanding waistline. I was going to have to get myself into shape. No matter how I felt about the whole thing. I was going to have to whip myself into shape. By (ugh!) ... dieting.

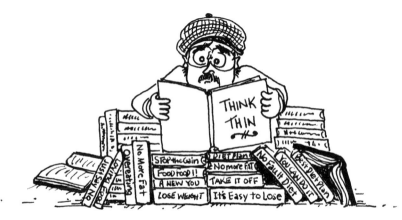

CHAPTER THREE
Deploying the Troops

So how was I going to do this dieting-thing? I mean, I was as lazy as a guy could be and still be considered somewhat ambulatory, and I did *love* to eat. So how could I possibly go about it and succeed?

My plan was really quite simple: I went out and purchased -- at a small fortune, I might add -- every book and pamphlet that had ever been written on the subject of dieting and specialized dieting plans. You name it, I bought it. And, because I anticipated many mental battles during my war on weight, I also bought a library of self-help and self-realization books to counterattack the urge to say to hell with everything. My philosophy was basically this: since I could no longer feed my stomach, the least I could do was feed my mind. A helluva trade-off at any rate.

I spent the next few days holed up in my room perusing my newly-acquired library and jotted down notes of comparison and differences between each of the program offerings. And all the while, I was shoveling mountains of junk food into my mouth like there was no tomorrow. Funny how that works.

What I discovered in my research was that, while each plan certainly seemed legitimate -- even potentially beneficial -- all of them were substantially flawed. From the perspective of Those Who Love To Eat. Here's why. Each diet plan that I reviewed practically forced me to fail at losing weight their way from the get-go by making me work hard at weighing all those yechy veggies and stuff they wanted to force-feed me, and by having me forsake the near and dear -- namely, most all those glorious foods that set my tastebuds aflutter with excitement and my tummy with gurgles of delight. And then -- get this -- the geniuses behind these programs wanted me to *exercise*. Fat chance.

There is one point that each of these books made that even I must agree upon, and it is this: before you consider pursuing any weight reduction plan -- including this one -- consult your physician or a healthcare professional. It is absolutely imperative.

And so, after weeks of mental fatigue and utter frustration, and having failed in my efforts to follow any of the prescribed programs for more than three days or so, this is precisely what *I* did.

*****

Herman Hepner had been my family's physician for most of my nineteen years, so it's pretty safe to say that he knew me and each member of my family -- physiologically speaking -- better than just about anyone. He had a manner that made you feel like you were the only patient he had, despite a waiting room that rivaled the population of, say, Rhode Island, at any given time. He was always careful to take the time to talk in depth about whatever ails his patients believed they had, and he always spoke candidly with each person he encountered in the examining rooms of his office. He was a man of great medical knowledge and infinite wisdom in the ways of human nature. To this day, I credit him for the success I achieved with this program. It was his candor about dieting and his encouragement that convinced me to give weight loss one last shot. His guidance and understanding were paramount in the development of what was to become the *Common Sense Approach to a Healthy Lifestyle*.

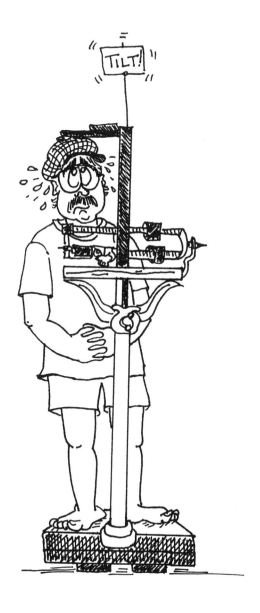

As attending physician to my father, Dr. Hepner was of course already completely aware of that situation. We spoke briefly concerning my father's condition and then I cut right to the chase, explaining to him that I was concerned about my health -- being so fat and out-of-shape, and all of that -- and wanted him to put me on a diet to save my life.

He nodded in agreement with everything I'd said and for the longest time he just sat there at his little table looking over my medical chart. Then he said point-blank, *"I don't believe in diet plans. And even if I did, you wouldn't follow it anyway."* I told you he was a man of infinite wisdom, didn't I?! The way he said it, so matter-of-factly, made my heart sink. I figured right then and there that I was just doomed to be fat and live a short, unfulfilled, bloated life as a result.

He did, however, agree with me about my need to lose weight or end up dead pretty quickly. So the program began inofficiously and unceremonially enough with a cursory physical examination that he performed right there in his office. It consisted of all my vital signs being checked for abnormalities of which there were none, fortunately. Then, with a sigh and not without trepidation, I stepped onto the gleaming white-and-silver Scales of Truth -- and injustice -- for the bane of a fat person's existence: the weigh-in. As it turned out, my weight was still within the accepted range handled by the office scale, sparing me the additional embarrassment and humiliation of having to trundle massively down to the local meat locker for a weigh-in there. Anyway, other than my substantial excess poundage that clung to my waist like a tremendous boa-constrictor, I passed the battery of tests with flying colors.

Upon completing the physical, we got down to the nitty-gritty and discussed exactly why I could not be faithful to any of those best-selling diet plans on the market. Fact of the matter was, I explained to the Good Doctor, I could not forsake the foods I loved to eat and I would not -- and probably *could not* -- make a point of exercising to the extent those programs told me I had to. Plain and simple.

What happened over the next fifteen or twenty minutes in that examination room was to change not only my attitude towards losing weight, but would have a profound -- and lasting -- effect on my life.

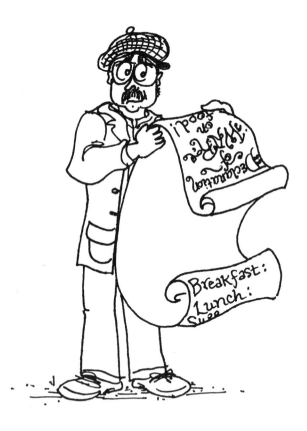

CHAPTER FOUR
Declaration of War

The premise of the plan that would become the *Common Sense Approach* that was developed during that office visit was really very basic. Those of us who love to eat and hate to exercise do not have the innate self-discipline to give up the food we enjoy, nor do we have the inherent determination and drive to start up exercising, so there is no way any of us can be completely true to the mandates of those diets. Well, guess what?! *YOU CAN HAVE YOUR CAKE AND EAT IT TOO*! Honest. That was the revelation that forever altered my life.

The principles of the *Common Sense Approach to a Healthy Lifestyle*, discussed in this chapter, not only permit you to eat whatever you want, but actually *encourage* you to. No way! you exclaim in total disbelief. Well, okay then. The *Common Sense Approach* **doesn't** encourage you. It *INSISTS* upon it! The beautiful thing is, you'll lose weight in a steady, healthy fashion that is conducive to keeping it off. In spite of yourself.

And what's more, under the *Approach* you aren't required or even *expected* to exercise any more than you would under normal circumstances. Nope. But you know what? Chances are, you'll discover that, as you design and implement your Personal Agenda under the *Approach*, your energy level will increase to the point that you'll actually begin to exercise more -- not because you have to, but because you'll *want* to!

By following the *Common Sense Approach*, I lost in excess of thirty pounds in just over a three month period. By the end of the fourth or fifth week, my energy level increased to the point where I actually *wanted* to get out and be more active than I was accustomed to being. About six weeks into the *Approach* my waistline had noticeably slimmed. And I hadn't given up a single item of food that I enjoyed eating. Not one. It was absolutely incredible.

*****

Any war can be won if the battle plan is well-conceived and implemented precisely. The *Common Sense Approach to a Healthy Lifestyle* is a carefully sculpted agenda and blueprint for success in fighting the war on overeating. By following the Attack Plans described in this chapter you will be waging a war against your waistline that you *can actually win* -- finally! You won't be forced to sacrifice a thing. Or exercise any more than you do right now. Promise.

There are no gimmicks or insane, wacko plots involved. If you approach the battle in the same fashion I did, you'll simply be making common sense decisions concerning your eating habits and ultimately, you'll find yourself sneaking around. Only this time you'll surprise yourself by sneaking in exercise rather than extra food. **The whole plan is simple and sensible.** The way things really ought to be.

With that said, let's grab our armor and ammunition and go to war!

*****

ATTACK PLAN I: VISIT YOUR PHYSICIAN AND GET A PHYSICAL

This could be the only common link between the *Common Sense Approach* and those run-of-the-mill diet plans, but it is absolutely imperative that you do it. If, like me, the only malady you suffer from is a voracious and insatiable appetite, then tip the scales and move on to the next Attack Plan.

However, if the examination reveals any abnormality -- no matter how inconsequential it may seem -- ask your physician to review the rest of the Attack Plans and offer alternative approaches without altering the basic spirit and philosophy of the *Approach*. In any event, remember that your health is at stake here and should never be compromised under any circumstances.

ATTACK PLAN II: WEIGH-IN AND SET A GOAL FOR YOURSELF

In order to achieve success, you must have a vision and set reasonable goals as a means of periodic measurement of your efforts. In the case of a fat person trying to lose weight, the measurement part is pretty simple: all we have to do is weigh ourselves. Now's as good a time as any. So pull out that bathroom scale and step up for the Moment of Truth. If you're like me and don't own a scale, do like I did and borrow one from somebody, okay?

Okay, you already got weighed at the doctor's office as part of your physical examination, but curiosity always gets the best of me. I want to see how big a difference there is between the doctor's scale and those household types that you buy at the store, don't you? Besides, unless your doctor is insisting upon closely monitoring your progress, there's really no point in putting down big bucks to visit his office just to weigh in. So, go on, step on to the platform and let the numbers whir before your eyes. Check it out. *Round and round she goes, where it stops nobody knows!* When it finally does stop, write the weight down on a piece of paper and put it in a safe place. I actually taped mine on the refrigerator door as a not-so-subtle reminder of my mission, but you do what you want with yours.

Now get rid of the scale. I've learned that the temptation to tip the scale too frequently when losing weight is a great one, and doing it more than once a month is an absolute no-no. Why? We of Hearty Girth don't want to do this diet thing to begin with, so we just naturally look for reasons to give up. And not seeing immediate results is the best reason of all to kill what little resolve we may have. Right?

Why, I bet if I asked point-blank whether or not you've tried to lose weight in the past and gave up because you couldn't resist the temptation of the Almighty Scale, nearly everyone of you would have to raise your hands. Am I right? Well, listen carefully. Immediate results ain't gonna happen. So do yourself a favor and get rid of your bathroom scale. If you weigh yourself too often, you'll only become despondent or angry or discouraged at the seeming lack of progress you're making. I know it for a fact.

The *Approach* is intentionally designed for weight loss over a prolonged period of time, so you are not going to lose ten pounds in a few days or even weeks, and weighing yourself daily or weekly will only serve to undermine the whole darn thing.

So get rid of that scale; besides, if you pitch it, there'll be one less thing lying around that you're apt to stub your toe on. If it means that much to you, have a friend take custody of it for awhile, or throw it away. I don't care. Just don't leave it somewhere convenient where it is liable to tempt you. Got it? Enough said.

Now that you know where you stand weight-wise and having consulted your friendly physician previously, you should have a firm idea of how much excess baggage you need to leave behind on the old weight-loss carousel to be at *your* ideal weight. What is the *ideal* weight, anyway? Good question. Remember those charts I mentioned a while back? Well, for what it's worth, they do merit *some* consideration when determining what ideal weight should be. Funny though, it seems these weight-chart people can't agree on things either, judging from recent articles I've read. Anyway, get your chubby little hands on one of those and look at it. Then throw it away. Your ideal weight will become self-apparent as you drop off the pounds. As you reach a certain point, you'll **know** that you're at the weight you are supposed to be. Maybe you'll look in the mirror and smile at that attractive, slender figure reflecting back; perhaps, it'll be as simple as a *feeling*. But you'll *know* when you've reached the ideal weight. One way or another. This, you can count on.

But of course for the sake of establishing a goal for yourself, you need guidance and direction in the how-much-weight-do-I-really-need-to-lose-to-be-fit-and-healthy decision, right? If your doctor was as insightful and helpful as mine was, he probably put his two-cents worth into the matter by telling you about where you should be weight-wise. What the heck, use that as your goal.

If you're still uncertain about whether you really have the gumption and wherewithal to see the *Approach* through, do this: find a full-length mirror that affords you some privacy. Get stark-naked and gaze at the reflection. What a sight, huh?

With that image in mind, close your eyes and imagine the leaner, more fit person you can be. Shoot, if it helps get the point across, visualize your favorite movie star or whomever else you might want to look like. Now, open your eyes. Which image makes you feel better? Seriously, folks, that visionary figure -- the lean, mean one -- can and *will* be you. Without a great deal of conscious effort on your part.

If you are like me, the realization that I had a ton (okay, it wasn't *quite* that much) of weight to lose was pretty damned shocking, not to mention, depressing. The *Common Sense Approach* is structured for about a ten-to-twelve pound loss each month, give or take a pound or two. So figure it will take you about one month for every ten pounds you want to trim off your weight. Go get your calendar and count off the number of months that is consistent with your intended weight loss. Put a great big star on that month. That's your V-W Day. **This is the day you declare your victory over weight!**

A note of caution: if you have an excessive amount of weight to lose -- excessive being over forty or fifty pounds -- I urge you to make a series of appointments with your physician or healthcare professional to allow for professional guidance and monitoring over the extended length of the *Approach.*

ATTACK PLAN III: PLAN YOUR PERSONAL AGENDA AND STRATEGIZE

Okay, if there really is a difficult part to the *Common Sense Approach*, this has got to be it. This Attack Plan requires you to analyze what -- and how much -- you eat over a period of a week. And when you eat it, which is important too. But, since this is heavy *mental* stuff, it's not like you're being asked to really *work*. No heavy labor stuff at all. But you do have to be *honest* about laying out your Personal Agenda, if you are seriously committed to the *Approach* and losing weight.

When you think about it, there is absolutely no reason not to be, since this little list you'll be compiling can be secreted away so that nobody ever sees it. And, if you just refuse to trust anybody at all -- or if you want to avoid the embarrassment of all those sidelong sneers and glib remarks by the skinny people of this world -- you can make mental notes if you have a really good memory. I don't recommend this method, however. This is really important stuff we're dealing with here -- the backbone of the whole body -- and it has to be accurate for the *Approach* to be beneficial. Personally, I found I was more successful plotting my strategy with notes in front of me than relying on my memory. Yes, I tried it *both* ways. You do what you like, though. It's your call.

If you're like me you will be really surprised at just how much food you consumed during your week of analysis (hey, don't confuse this form of analysis with that kind offered by those high-priced, glitzy, mind-game therapist-types, okay?). Once you know how much you eat and when you eat it, the strategy is quite simple: over the course of the next few weeks, you are going to cut down -- *not out* -- what you've been accustomed to eating.

I can just hear the whiners of the group now: "Oh God! I'm going to be *sooo* hungry I couldn't possibly live through all the pain and suffering of cutting down." Or some such nonsense like that. Fact of the matter is, you will be a *little* hungry at first, but it's not as bad as it sounds. Trust me, I've been there, remember? You will be hungry, at least for two or three or four days as you adjust your eating habits. But it won't be as nasty a hunger as you may think.

The whole key to success is to **reduce your consumption** based on your initial analysis, but to do it *gradually*.

For example, if you discover -- as I did -- that you have a real tendency to help yourself to three or four generous servings at dinner time, during the first week on the *Common Sense Approach* you will strive to eliminate *just one* of those helpings. Then as your stomach is getting used to that whole idea, you'll begin toying with cutting back on the *size* of the portion you dish out to yourself.

In other words, by the end of Week One you'll be eating two or three servings (or whatever is one less than your analysis) instead of three or four, and at the same time, rather than taking a *mammoth* glob of, say, those mashed potatoes along with everything else being served, you will reduce it to, maybe, just a glob.

I'll explain this in greater detail a little later, so if you don't quite understand the principle yet, don't worry -- it may cause you to eat a gigantic bag of your favorite cookies which would be somewhat counterproductive.

Anyway, the strategy phase of this Attack Plan is to gradually shrink your serving portions while, at the same time, shrinking your need (or is it want?) without sacrificing any of your favorite foods. Now, what you will actually be doing is developing that once-elusive concept of **willpower** which the *Common Sense Approach* defines as, "the act of extending your arms to the edge of the dinner table and thrusting one's body in an opposite direction, away from said dinner table, despite the continued presence of foodstuffs clearly visible to the naked eye, and the magnetic attraction emanating from said foodstuffs."

One of the flaws that I discovered with conventional, commercial diet plans was the insistence that the dieter exercise willpower immediately like it was something that came in a bottle and was ready-to-serve. Well, it don't just happen, folks. What these diets fail to consider is that we People of Excessive Weight more than likely got to where we are -- which is to say, overweight -- because for whatever reason, we never could quite figure out this willpower thing. Personally, I was always inclined to believe that genetics entered into my weight problems somewhere along the line, but it probably didn't.

Anyway, this willpower thing -- or rather, the *lack* of it in us Chubby Ones -- is a concept that seems to fly right over the heads of all those people who put together those conventional programs. What has to be done is simple. We have to coax ourselves **gradually** -- so we *can get used to the idea* of eating less -- not just jump right into it. The insistence that we conjure up enough willpower to spring into and follow the principles of these other weight loss methods has disaster and failure written all over it. The *Common Sense Approach to a Healthy Lifestyle* addresses that potential by teaching you how to build up willpower over the course of three, even four or five, weeks. We do it *gradually*. The *Approach* holds your hand, if you will, and guides you along the primrose path to the Wonderful World of Willpower. The hand-holding works. It helped me; it can and will help you.

ATTACK PLAN IV: THE POT O' GOLD AT THE END OF THE RAINBOW

You've been asked to do a lot over the first three Attack Plans. And especially with the last one, you have been requested to put forth considerable effort, not to mention, having to plan on cutting back your level of consumption.

Well, fair's fair. It really is time you get something in return for your efforts so far. This is the fun part.

Another flaw I realized with those dastardly diet plans was that while they expected me to give up all this food that I loved to eat, while they wanted me to measure out and eat a whole lot of those God-awful yechy veggies, and while they insisted that I get up off my fat duff and exercise, the only incentive they provided was so damned abstract and so far down the road that I couldn't possibly grasp the point of it all. So I couldn't help but become discouraged and frustrated with the whole thing.

Heck, I wound up cheating after about two or three days and finally abandoned the stupid plan altogether in less than a week. So much for losing weight the old-fashioned way.

The *Common Sense Approach* is just that: good old common sense. And, because I am essentially lazy and anti-diet by nature, I needed to have an incentive that meant something -- something a bit more instantly-gratifying than just the end-result weight loss -- if I was to achieve my lofty goal of losing thirty-odd pounds or so. Thus, while most diets are long-range, long-term in their thinking and process, the *Approach* shrinks and compresses the concept into week-long sections -- about as long as my diet-related attention span -- and provides a real honest-to-goodness incentive that you can sink your teeth into. Literally.

Stop and think for a moment. What is absolutely your favorite treat? Mine's ice cream, and lots of it. I swear I can't live without it. I would imagine you believe the same thing about your favorite treat. Well, common sense told me that, unless I found some sort of *avante-garde* diet plan that incorporated lots of ice cream in its regimen, I was destined to slip and slide and fall from its good graces.

Unless I got my ice cream fix through the marvels of some outrageous new diet scheme, I was going to lose the Battle of the Bulge. Before I could ever really begin. No doubt about it.

Bottom line here is this: I reviewed plenty of diets and none let me eat ice cream on a regular basis -- if *ever* -- so I sort of just had to cheat and eat it whenever I wanted, and because I wasn't losing any weight, I got discouraged and eventually just dropped out of the program. I mean, why follow a diet plan to gain weight when you can forsake it altogether and accomplish the same thing? Hardly makes any sense to diet that way. For that matter, I believe it doesn't make sense to diet in any way. So there.

The *Common Sense Approach* is designed to allow for that mental struggle thing with your favorite treat. **YOU CAN EAT IT**. Unheard of? Absolutely! Revolutionary? Hardly. It's just good old common sense.

Let me ask you this: would you work at a job you really hated (or loved, for that matter) without accepting a paycheck? I doubt it. And there is no reason under the sun to forego your favorite treat just because you're trying to lose weight. Rather, **your treat is a pot of gold at the end of the rainbow**.

If you faithfully follow the strategy you set up in Attack Plan III, you should be rewarded for your honest effort at the end of the week. Just like when you're working. That *is* what dieting is to us, isn't it? A tremendous amount of work. Okay, I can hear the so-called experts out there saying things like, "What keeps a person from cheating on the *Approach* during the week and rewarding himself anyway?" or "That approach won't work in getting people to lose weight. Too much temptation and a gigantic loophole in the concept and thinking." Maybe so.

The only way I can respond to those would-be critics is by citing my own personal experience. I found that most People of Excessive Weight really want to weigh less -- for both personal and health reasons -- but they are too easily tempted by the Fates of Food and the siren songs of sumptuous aromas that waft enticingly from the Caverns of Great Things To Eat. Because the *Common Sense Approach* gets to the heart of the matter -- *the appetite* -- in a far less dramatic fashion, it is easier for the participant to stay the course and resist temptation. And, that's what it's really all about, this weight loss game. The subtle changes in your eating habits, implemented early in the *Approach*, are designed to encourage success.

I found that during the initial week I had no difficulty being faithful to the Personal Agenda I had planned; after all, there was the matter of a reward for my efforts just a scant, few days away. The further I got into my strategy, my appetite and the thoughts of a little more food were suppressed sufficiently enough that just a quick flash of that reward -- in my case, a half-pint of my favorite ice cream -- diverted my attention just long enough for the urge to cheat to slither away.

But hey, no one's perfect. I did discover that the one time I did cheat on the *Approach* during the week, I couldn't bring myself to order the ice cream. I mean, I walked right up to the girl at the counter, slapped the money down, but I just couldn't get the words out of my mouth. Honest. You see, I am basically an honest person and besides, even if I wasn't, the last person I would ever want to cheat would be myself. I truly believe that people who are Willpower-Challenged investigating the *Common*

Sense Approach feel the same way. To thine own self be true. Words to live by. And to lose weight by.

Anyway, Attack Plan IV is simply about setting a reward for yourself. It is an essential ingredient to succeeding in the Battle of the Bulge. After a week of being completely faithful to the strategy of the *Approach*, treat yourself to something really tasty. I mean, really *splurge* with it. You earned it. As hard as it may be to believe, this method of treating yourself *weekly* really does work. I couldn't have succeeded without it.

ATTACK PLAN V: EFFECTING THE STRATEGY
There are certain foods that we all know we should avoid. It seems every time you watch a news program on television or read the evening newspaper, some new study has come out with still *another* kind of food that we should forget about. Holy cow! The list of *no-no* foods seems practically endless in length. Shoot, eventually the only foods those research people will allow us to eat are those veggie-type stuff. Yech! Don't get me wrong, I'm not condemning any of these reports. After all, these lab-coated guys have spent many years and big bucks researching all this, so they *must* know of what they speak.

So, as I mentioned, there are certain foods we all know we should avoid. The problem We of Chubby Girth have is that we just do not *want* to. We know what we like, and we'll usually eat it.

Most, if not all, diet plans preach from a self-righteous pulpit that you absolutely, positively must cut out this food or that food to lose weight. The *Common Sense Approach* says, with its hearty, cynical laugh, "Bullpucky!" It just ain't so. **You don't have to deny yourself a single, solitary thing**. What you really need to do is *moderate* your consumption of those nasty, good-tasting foods that every diet condemns.

In that office visit with Dr. Hepner so many years ago, he provided me with a comprehensive list of foods that I needed to moderate if I were to seriously attempt to lose weight:

•Potatoes	•Corn	•Peas
•Whole Milk	•Ice Cream	•Bread
•Cheese	•Butter	•Eggs
•Baked Goods	•Candy	

For those health-conscious believers in the Purveyors of Unpleasant News As It Relates To Eating, I *could* say that the list of *no-no* foods went on and on. But I won't. Why? Because, quite honestly, that was it. Quite a lengthy list of foods, huh?

The Kind Doctor just rattled off those few items and explained that everyone should monitor their consumption of starchy foods. He added that, if I made an honest effort to control my binges on these particular items, I would have no trouble losing weight. He was, as they say, right as rain.

But the important thing to remember is that the operative word here is **moderate** -- not give up or cut out. I could handle that. For the record, I love every single item on that list and if he had told me to give up even one of them, I probably would have found another doctor, or just resigned myself to being a blimp. No way would I be willing to sacrifice any of the foods that comprised the bulk of my diet. Besides, everybody knows you can't teach an old dog new tricks. Right?

*****

So how do you go about moderating your consumption? Well, guess what? If you've followed the Attack Plans up to now you've pretty much already outlined how you're going to do it. But to carefully outline a program and to really implement the change are two vastly different matters, right? Wrong. There is *no secret* to it. There is *no mystery*. All you have to do from here on is *gradually* reduce the number of portions you help yourself to, while *gradually* reducing the size of the servings you take. Sound familiar? Before you know it, you will be eating far less than you started out eating.   And don't forget that marvelous reward at the end of the week for having done so well!

To illustrate how simple implementation of change can be, I will use my own Personal Agenda as an example. The premise here is that, as in my case, if you are shooting to lose roughly thirty pounds, your Agenda should reflect the full extent of your change -- that's the reduction in consumption -- by the end of the third week. If you are looking to lose forty pounds or so, your Agenda needs to stretch to a fourth week; with fifty-plus pounds, your reduction in consumption should extend to five or six weeks. And so on. In the case of extreme amounts of weight to be lost, the Agenda should be reviewed by your physician or healthcare professional.

The point of the *Common Sense Approach* is that you should modify your eating habits gradually, with the least amount of resistance from your stomach and your mind. And it will be far more difficult to do that in the early days and weeks of the Agenda -- as you retrain your mind and begin shrinking your stomach -- so bite off only what you can comfortably chew early on. It's real simple. Let your common sense be your guide. **Modify *gradually*.**

But however you go about changing your eating habits, don't get carried away with the old *doing-too-much-too-soon* syndrome because it simply will not work. You may lose lots and lots of weight quickly, but you could also seriously affect your health doing it. Or, you could end up doing great that way -- which is to say, *starving* yourself -- for three or four days and then, all of a sudden you will get hit with this tremendous urge to binge and you'll start eating. And eating. And eating. So perish the thought of the instant weight loss. It just won't work.

How can I be so sure? Hey, I've been there, remember? I'm not some skinny guy in a white lab coat who knows these things *theoretically*. I'm one of you. I've tried everything. Every way. Believe me, theory didn't work. Quick-fix didn't work. The reality is that until I followed my common sense, I was fat -- real fat. So heed my words, here: don't rush into it. **Modify your appetite *gradually*.** It will work.

Okay then. Let's review my Personal Agenda, shall we? We'll peek first at a synopsis of the list I made from the week of analysis, then we will outline the modification process.

BREAKFAST
I'd generally begin my day with a hearty breakfast; after all, the experts always advised us that it was the *most important* meal of the day. So typically, I would eat three or four peanut butter sandwiches on toast -- that's six or eight *slices* of bread -- or two bowls of cereal and one or two sandwiches, washed down with two or three tumblers of ice-cold milk. There were days when I opted for three or four fried eggs and three or four slices of toast smothered in butter. That

was when I was thinking more health-consciously, though.

LUNCH

My eating habits at lunch time were pretty routine. I'd prepare two sandwiches of virtually any processed meat -- smothered in mayonnaise or some other garnishment -- and slice up a lot of cheese, and add a generous portion of potato chips on the side. I'd generally consume at least one twelve-ounce soda, but on occasion I'd treat myself to a second one. On those days when I really felt like treating myself, I'd take myself to lunch at the local diner and feast on whatever met my fancy. A bowl of chili. A couple of cheeseburgers. Maybe even one substantial serving of my personal favorite, macaroni and cheese. Mind you, this was *in addition to* eating my packed lunch.

DINNER

My appetite at dinner was always voracious. I would eat at least three, if not four, *tremendous* helpings of everything served. Mountains of potatoes awash in a sea of gravy; enormous portions of meat; and, lots and lots of peas or corn, those being the only vegetables I liked. It usually required two or three large glasses of whole milk to satisfy my thirst at dinner. And, oh yes, if a dessert was prepared (as it routinely was), I would insist on eating two generous helpings of it.

SNACKS

Here's the really great part. My snacking was virtually non-stop during the day and night. In the morning, I'd munch on a sweet roll and drink plenty of milk; for added energy in the afternoon, I could almost always be seen with a candy bar in one hand and a soda in the other; and, in the evening while watching television, I'd eat a bowl of ice cream -- usually four or five heaping scoops -- or a dozen cookies or so dunked in a glass of milk. If dessert had, in fact, been served at dinner, you can bet I cleaned it out that night. Sometimes, if I was really hungry, a sandwich or two would precede the snack and, no matter what, I always drank at least one sixteen-ounce soda every evening.

Please remember that this is just a synopsis of my analysis week. The actual list was kept very accurately, recording the time of day that I ate and how much I shoved into my mouth at one sitting. I chose the synopsis format for this book simply because to use my actual method of logging the things I ate would have made this book about the size of a standard encyclopedia.

Looking back, I confess that I am truly shocked and appalled at the amount of food I was consuming in a day's time. Yes, I am gravely ashamed of myself. But those are the indisputable facts and it certainly is a graphic illustration of why I was grotesquely overweight back then.

*****

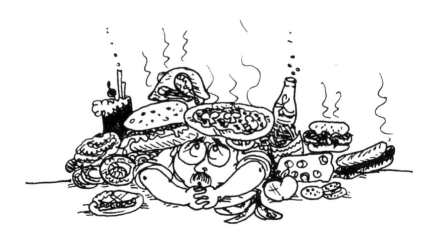

Now for the *Common Sense Approach* to reducing your food consumption. Again, the number of weeks you need to implement this strategy is strictly based upon the amount of weight you wish to lose. In my case, the goal was just a little over thirty pounds, so my Agenda was set at three weeks.

And I'll confess to another thing right now: during those first three or four days, it was real tough to follow through with the program, what with hunger pangs pounding away at the insides of my stomach. But each time I was ready to concede and give in to those dastardly urges, I closed my eyes and pictured how great that ice cream -- every sumptuous, delicious bite of the half-pint -- was going to taste at the end of the week. It managed to console me. Sweet inspiration, as it were.

WEEK ONE

BREAKFAST
The three or four peanut butter sandwiches dwindled to two by the third morning of Week One. When I opted for the healthier repast of fried eggs, my limit was three -- scrambled -- with no more than two pieces of toast to complement them. I still drank milk, but no more than one glass, compensating with coffee or water instead. During that first week when I ate cereal, it was still two bowls, sans the sandwich chaser.

LUNCH
The week started with the unceremonial dispatch of the chips and cheese from my lunchtime repast. The third day of Week One marked the trimming of the second sandwich to but a mere half, so that by the end of the week I was eating but one whole sandwich as

my luncheon mainstay. I also forced myself to drink only one soda, no matter what. And on those occasions when I felt like treating myself by drifting into the diner for a hot meal, I eliminated my prepacked lunch by casting it into the trash on my way out the door. It was a tough thing to do, but I did it -- without remorse.

DINNER

Common sense led me to believe that this meal would be the most difficult to alter so I had to really plan my attack carefully. I began the week by reducing the *size* of my portions, then on the fourth day I made the plunge by killing the urge to help myself to more than three servings. On the sixth and seventh days, I limited myself to but two helpings of the dinner -- just to *mentally* prepare myself for what lay ahead. I drank milk but would substitute water for a second glass. As for any dessert served, I permitted myself a very substantial portion, but only *one*.

SNACKS

Where -- and *what* -- to cut out! I essentially attempted to mentally trick myself for the first few days. I substituted several cookies for that one morning sweet roll. The familiar *the-more-the-merrier number* set to food. I started out giving myself eight small cookies and reduced the number by one every other day. Perhaps the most difficult task I faced that first week was my decision to eliminate that afternoon candy bar -- my energy booster. I settled for the rush of an ice-cold soda, drinking lots of water to stave off the midday demon hunger pangs. Another little trick I utilized was to chew a lot of gum to keep my mouth busy as I attempted to trim the candy from my snacking routine. It really worked. As for the evening snack, I made the decision right away to relegate the nightly soda to an every-other-night treat -- it served as a mini-reward for doing good. What I discovered, rather interestingly, over the course of the week was that the nighttime snacking was less of an issue than I had anticipated. Beginning with a bunch of cookies coupled with the leftover dessert, by the end of the week I'd managed to cut back to one or the other, but never both. Again, water became a very good substitute for my desire to constantly snack on food.

Oh yes, I did eat a half-pint of my favorite ice cream at the end of the week.

I didn't just automatically knock down the consumption level. Each day, little-by-little, the subtle changes were undertaken so the plan was stretched out *over the course of the whole week* ... I knew going in each week how much I had eaten the *previous* one, and I envisioned where I wanted to be -- consumption-wise -- by the end of that week. The modification was *gradual*. And as a result, the fits of hunger and yearnings associated with it, minimal.

*****

WEEK TWO

BREAKFAST

Something extraordinary occurred early in Week Two: my appetite had declined dramatically. The two peanut butter sandwiches gave way to no more than one-and-a-half sandwiches by the second day. My goal of eating only one sandwich by the end of the week was accomplished by Day Three. On those occasions when I elected to eat cereal instead of toast

-- my idea of balancing my diet, by the way -- I was amazed to discover that one bowl more than filled me up.

LUNCH

On the fourth day of the week, I leaped into action by substituting a generous portion of cottage cheese and a hard-boiled egg for my beloved sandwich, and elected to drink a small amount of milk instead of the soda. For a couple of days, I felt I needed to eat a half a sandwich, but by the end of the week, the mainstay of my midday feast was the cottage cheese, with sliced peaches to break up the blandness, and a hard-boiled egg. I resisted the temptation to take myself to lunch at the local restaurant, instead playing the mind-game routine by *envisioning* a hearty repast while scarfing down my cottage cheese. It wasn't perfect, mind you, but it got me through.

DINNER

Over the course of the week, I concentrated on further reducing the size of the portions I served myself. By mid-week I was controlling my appetite with two *average* servings of the dinner, although I would often times bypass seconds on everything but the main dish. And of course I still had a very healthy helping of any dessert that was served.

SNACKS

Week Two was one full of surprises and phenomena, dietarily speaking. The urge for substantial evening snacks was dramatically diminished by the third or fourth day of Week Two. Whenever it was overwhelming, I'd generally munch on three or four cookies with a small glass of milk to chase them down, or have an *average-sized* portion of the evening's dessert. What I discovered was that on those nights when I drank my sixteen-ounce soda, no other snack was really necessary to quell the urges. Daytime snacks were virtually in the *Smithsonian* -- like other significant matters of history. I had little need for a morning snack; and, in the afternoon I would drink a twelve-ounce soda. That was it.

And because I'd been such a good boy and followed my Personal Agenda faithfully, I ate a half-pint of my favorite ice cream at the end of the week.
*****

WEEK THREE

Week Three represented the summit of the mountain for me, as the last week of your Personal Agenda will for you. Once you reach the summit, it's all downhill from there. No longer will the urges haunt you and tug at your tummy. You will have significantly diminished your level of consumption, ideally to an *average* one. You'll find your appetite -- and your stomach -- shrinking. And the really great thing is: you have been able to enjoy all those great foods you always have, *including* your weekly reward. Without *it* being dangled in front of me, especially in the early going, I would not have made it to this point.

BREAKFAST
From three or four sandwiches at the outset, I had now altered my habits to where I sometimes was eating as little as one slice of toast generously smeared with butter, and a couple of glasses of milk. There were a couple of days during Week Three when I actually *skipped* breakfast altogether. What I discovered was that I would only eat when I was *hungry*, and not simply because the food was there in

front of me. A subtle, yet significant, change in my eating habits.

LUNCH
By the end of the week, my lunch was consistently cottage cheese with an occasional hard-boiled egg. Once during the week I treated myself to a soda instead of relying on milk as my beverage of choice. I also went out to the diner one day for lunch because -- get this -- I craved a salad. I still have a difficult time with that one, but it's true.

DINNER
Starting out the week I was pretty much helping myself to two servings of everything, although I had a hard time finishing that second round. By the end of Week Three I had successfully reduced my portions to one average serving. And with that eaten, I'd often find myself contentedly patting or rubbing my stomach. As far as dessert goes, you should know by now that I'm the type of guy who just cannot say no. Everytime dessert was offered, I gladly accepted it. No question. No guilt.

SNACKS
Other than my soda every other evening and an occasional craving for sweets, the urge to snack was pretty much out of the picture. If a quick flash in my mind of that half-pint of ice cream didn't subdue the craving, I'd eat two or three cookies. That was it. Another interesting personal phenomenon occurred during Week Three as well. I actually began munching on fruit as a substitute for the really sweet, sugary stuff. Near the end of the week I got a real strong urge to eat a banana, so I did. Without feeling really weird, even. Ultimately, bananas and apples

became part and parcel to my Personal Agenda. There's not really much to say about my propensity for daytime snacking, other than it was virtually nonexistent. Other than an occasional soda or an apple, I just never felt the urge. Or the *need*.

Yes, of course, since I'd been a true-blue follower of my Agenda and the *Approach* for the whole week, I peacefully devoured that half-pint of ice cream -- my just dessert for my efforts.

*****

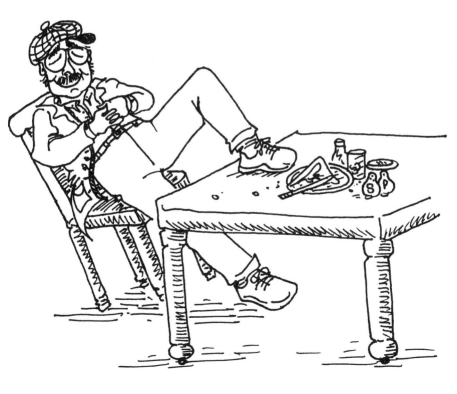

SUMMARY

So there you have a peak at my Personal Agenda over the initial three weeks of the *Common Sense Approach*. The same concept should be instituted as you plan out your initial Agenda. That is to say, you should be deliberate in adjusting your eating habits, taking care not to rush the reduction process.

If you do, you will ultimately fall into the same kind of trappings that are present in all those diet plans that just don't seem to work, and you'll be setting yourself up for a mega-fall. **Make sure the adjustment in your eating habits is *gradual* and *methodical*.** Otherwise, you will be tempted to cheat and defeat the principle of the *Common Sense Approach.*

ATTACK PLAN VI: TIPS TO GET YOU THROUGH THE STRUGGLES

Okay, maybe I have painted a pretty rosy picture, or maybe you're just not convinced that the *Common Sense Approach* really can work for you. I admit, it's a pretty whacko concept to promote a weight loss program that lets you eat everything you always have and gives you a sweet-tasting reward each week to do it. But, the fact of the matter is, folks, I had tried lots and lots of times to lose weight by conventional means without any success. Why? Because they all expected too much from me too soon. When in my frustration I went and spoke with the Good Doctor about losing weight, he essentially was telling me to use my judgment about things. *He wanted me to quit working so damned hard at dieting and just do what felt right.*

During the initial stages of trying to figure out what made sense to me, I fell into some typical traps, had to take a few steps back to evaluate the situation, and then make a few adjustments. In other words, the *Common Sense Approach to a Healthy Lifestyle* was developed through trial-and-error, and this book is the result of those efforts -- what worked best to help me, a lazy anti-diet Person of Excessive Weight, beat down the foe and lose weight I never could before.

It wasn't always a piece of cake (no pun intended) and I had those moments when I could have given in but didn't. Why? Because I let my common sense lead me through the war. With a little common sense guiding you along through the storm, you're never completely alone. I beat the battle and you can too.

Since I know you will go through many of the same things I did, Attack Plan VI is designed to offer a few modest suggestions and reminders to help you get by those Demon Temptations which, by the way, you shouldn't confuse with that terrific Motown singing group from the 60s and 70s. They were great, these demon ones aren't so hot. Anyway, here they are (the suggestions, not the Temptations), in no particular order.

IF IT DOESN'T MAKE SENSE, DON'T DO IT. This is probably the *Cardinal Rule* of the *Common Sense Approach*, if there is one. Think about what you are doing at any given point -- especially when facing obstacles or doubts -- and if it doesn't make sense to you, then forget it. Early in your assault against the Demons of Desire, you are going to have to listen to a lot of rumblings and grumblings from your stomach complaining in its inimitable way about the lack of nutritional substance it is being fed. Ignore it. Listen, instead, to what your *mind* is telling you. Pay attention to your common sense. It will never steer you wrong. That's why this book is called what it's called.

AS YOU BEGIN MODIFYING YOUR APPETITE BY REDUCING YOUR CONSUMPTION LEVELS, EAT SLOWLY AND SAVOR EVERY BITE. Take your time eating, especially in the early stages of your Personal Agenda. Eating slowly has a way of tricking your mind *and* your stomach into believing you're eating more. I don't profess to know why. I just know it works that way.

VISUALIZE THE POT O' GOLD AT THE END OF THE RAINBOW. What are you to do when that constant thumping and yearning in your stomach escalates to the point of driving you to the fringe of madness? Relax. Close your eyes. Visualize that very special pot of gold at the end of the rainbow. It's not *that* far from your reach. I can't begin to explain how critical it was for me to know that I could indulge myself at the end of a long, trying week of fighting the Demons. It kept me focused and on track.

GIVE YOURSELF A MINI-REWARD EVERY OTHER NIGHT TO KEEP YOU ON TRACK DURING YOUR WEEK-LONG STRUGGLES. If you just do not believe you are capable of lasting a whole week -- after all, that's *seven* twenty-four hour days -- do what I did: cut out one of your routine evening snacks. Then give it back to yourself every other day. If it's food rather than drink, reduce the normal serving to half as much. Nothing wrong with treating yourself in a mini-fashion; you've been working hard at this diet-thing, and you deserve a break. Just remember that this is a give-and-take situation. Give yourself a pat-on-the-back, but make it smaller. There's something far grander waiting for you at the end of the week, you know.

AS YOU WAGE THE BATTLE WITH SNACKING, TRY SUBSTITUTING GREAT TASTING FRUIT LIKE BANANAS AND PEACHES FOR COOKIES, CAKES, AND PIES. As I reduced my consumption of snack foods, I would occasionally experiment with fruit to see if my body could actually learn to accept unconditionally -- without fear of rejection -- *natural* sweeteners rather than stuff which amounted to nothing more than compressed sugar. Guess what? Not only did my body accept this fruit thing, but fact of the matter is, I was completely surprised at how great it tasted. What I discovered was that one banana arrested the hunger pangs and tasted just as good as those cookies I was accustomed to eating, but with a lot less calories to worry about. Things like sliced peaches or pears, apples, and canned fruit cocktail were personal favorites, and helped change my snacking habits. And they managed to satisfy my cravings for sweets. Hey, if you're concerned about what your friends may say if they catch you snacking on fruit, just munch on it in the dark, late at night when no one's apt to drop in on you. It'll be worth it, believe me.

TAKE IT SLOWLY AND DELIBERATELY. I emphasized this earlier in the chapter, but it is so important, it merits special attention here. Don't be too hasty in attempting to lose weight. Rome wasn't built in a day, you know. Look at it this way: you didn't get to be excessively overweight in a day or two, or even weeks. It took months, maybe longer, to become a blimp. So why would you believe you could knock it off quickly? You were successful gaining the weight over an extended period of time, so it stands to reason that you will be successful losing it in the same fashion. Okay, maybe that isn't a rational argument, but you serve no good by trying to take the weight off quickly. None. Nada. Zip. The *Approach* is designed to reduce deliberately. The problem with diet plans is that they expect you to change your eating habits *overnight*. Well, I don't know about you, but that's not something I could ever do successfully. Take your time and do it right. Be patient. Do it *gradually*.

DON'T FIGHT THE FEELING TO GET OUT AND EXERCISE MORE WHEN YOUR ENERGY LEVEL INCREASES (AND IT WILL). I was amazed at how quickly my energy level increased once I began the *Approach*. The amount of energy increase seemed directly proportional to the amount of the consumption decrease. The less I ate, the more energetic and ambitious I became. So I got out and walked when I could have driven. Things like that. Just don't fight the feeling, okay? The exercise will help keep you directed on your mission. Promise.

AVOID THE PITFALLS OF BEING IDLE. Idle minds are the Devil's workshop, right? Don't get caught up in feeding your idle time or boredom with food. Feed it, instead, with games -- either mental or physical -- or some sort of recreational activity. Just don't eat for the sake of eating. Call a friend and get away from the temptation. Do whatever it takes. This is extremely important advice, *especially in the early going.* You are going to experience tremendous urges that, without diversion, could beat you down and cause you to give in. Don't do it. Find someone -- or something -- to keep you busy.

*****

There you go. A few tips and reminders that will help keep you directed in your efforts to effect the various Attack Plans we've discussed and get you on your way to losing the weight you never thought you could. And winning the Battle of the Bulge. Everybody's different, I know, but if you put your heart into finding your pot o' gold at the end of the rainbow every week, if you focus your mind on your mission, and if you follow the lead of your common sense, you'll be able to eat what you want, strip off the pounds, and become more involved in recreational activities -- and *life*. And, believe me, exercising for fun is a hell of a lot better (and easier) than doing it because you have to. The keys to success with the *Common Sense Approach* are simply to reward yourself for your efforts each week, and relying on your common sense to do it.

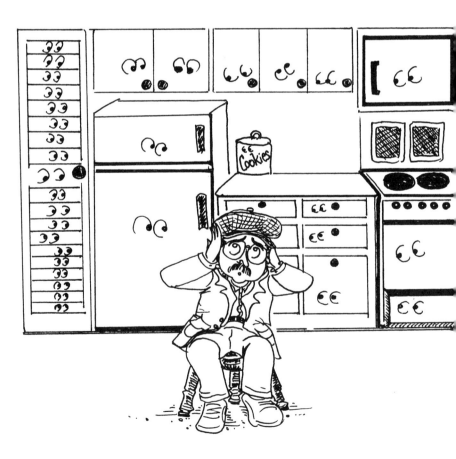

CHAPTER FIVE
The Battle of the Bulge

After toying with several diet plans for a number of weeks, and after a few false starts with the development of the *Common Sense Approach*, my personal Battle of the Bulge began in earnest in early 1971. With a fresh concept in mind, I set out to wage the war, somewhat dispirited from my past troubled campaigns against a rather formitable foe -- my expanding waistline.

Relying on the Attack Plans I had developed and, armed with nothing more than a renewed determination, I marched blindly into the fray. My goal: thirty-plus pounds and five inches from my waist.

The first four days were pure hell. No other way to describe it. As I trimmed my consumption level from three or four servings down to a mere two, hunger pangs battered at the pit of my stomach with an unrelenting pugilistic force. I prowled around the house dodging the incoming missiles of snack food being hurtled in my direction from the bunkers of the kitchen cabinets and the refrigerator.

Those initial nights were restless ones, spent tossing and turning, as dreams led me through enchanted forests of hot fudge sundaes and ice cream sodas; of chocolate layer cakes and hot apple pies. Mountains of mashed potatoes tipped with melting butter were beckoning from beyond wide rivers of giblet gravy drifting lazily at the forest's edge. Despondent and under seige, I peered through cream-puff clouds and spotted a ray of hope: a rainbow, at the end of which was a pot o' gold.

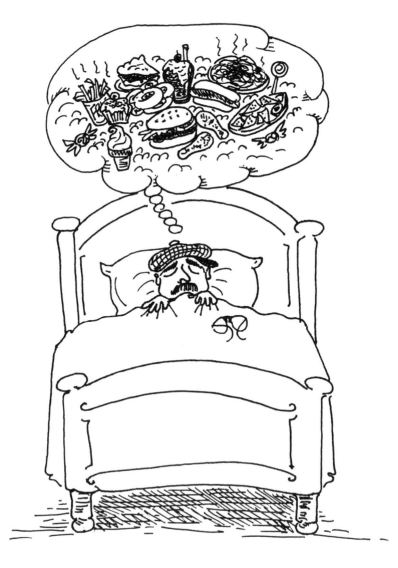

I suffered my first casualty of war on the fifth day. A battalion of sweets, commandeered by a tremendous chocolate cupcake, resorted to guerilla war tactics and ambushed my camp, mining its perimeter. A piece of chocolate layer cake besieged me and took me prisoner. Torture and humiliation ensued.

Left to my own devices and, relying on common sense alone, I escaped from my captors disguised as an immense Hostess Snowball. With but minor injuries to my pride, despite the deplorable conditions and my waning morale, I regrouped with a vow to return to battle with renewed vigor.

For three weeks the war waged on, small victories claimed and celebrated with the ceremonial raising of the Baskin-Robbins banner each week, as I savored the view from the summit. It was near the middle of that third week that I began feeling confident that the enemy lines were weakening. The counterattacks were less frequent; their force, less dynamic. Victory was mine for the claiming. And, as sweet as a cinamon roll fresh from the baker's oven.

*****

After the first month of following the *Common Sense Approach*, I stepped on the scales for the first time: I had lost eight pounds even though I had spent the better part of three weeks rearranging my eating habits. I had hardly begun the war, but was already eight pounds lighter. And what had I sacrificed? I'd eaten everything that had been prepared, treated myself to a half-gallon of my favorite ice cream, and here I was losing weight.

It was the second month that my friends began commenting on my slimming waistline and the *Approach* was essentially second-nature to me. There were no more longing looks at the leftovers on the table; rather, I'd find myself contentedly patting my stomach after eating a meager portion -- by my accustomed standards -- of the repast.

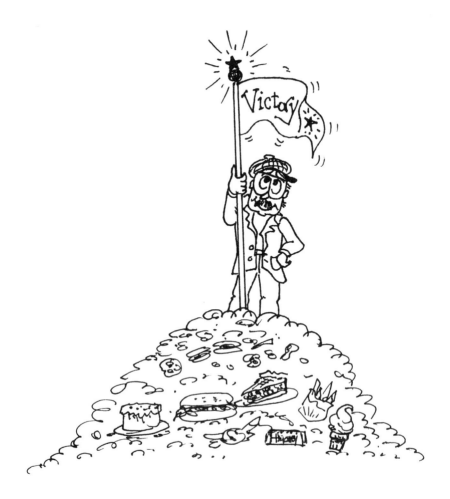

It was sometime shortly before my second weigh-in that it occurred to me that I was actually eating more fruit than baked goods. It was absolutely astounding!

What's more, I slipped on a pair of slacks that had once been ever so snug-fitting and discovered that they still didn't fit well at all. Except this time, they were way too big! When I took those slacks to be altered, they had to be taken in at the waist *over three inches*! Man, I was so stoked! I felt like I had finally *arrived*. My lifestyle and physical looks were actually changing unbeknownst to me. Pretty amazing stuff.

Tipping the scales at the end of Month Two, I was surprised to discover that I had lost another thirteen pounds. Twenty-one pounds in two months. Friends telling me how great I looked. Clothes having to be taken *in* to fit me. And another half-gallon of my favorite ice cream devoured without guilt.

With the changes going on in my lifestyle, I discovered differences in my attitude and approach to life in general. No longer looking or feeling frumpy, my enthusiasm returned and my energy was recharged. I bought new clothes; I walked places instead of driving my car. I socialized and became involved in recreational programs. In other words, **I got a life**. It was truly exciting. And, I was still scarfing down a half-pint of ice cream each and every week as a reward for sticking to the *Common Sense Approach to a Healthy Lifestyle*.

My third weigh-in confirmed that I had succeeded in making my goal. I'd lost another ten pounds, making a total loss over a three month period thirty-one pounds. Phenomenal, to say the least, for a guy who had all but given up on diets and exercise.

Truth of the matter was, the *Common Sense Approach* wasn't *really* a diet -- in the conventional sense, anyway. Or at least it didn't *feel* like one, and that was really important.

Hey, you need to keep in mind that so much of the battle to lose weight is **IN THE MIND**, and believing that the *Approach* wasn't like a real diet -- whether or not it really is does not enter into it -- helped conquer that vast wasteland of the mind.

*****

There wasn't a flaw in the *Approach* that I could find in those initial three months. I ate well. I ate what I wanted and always treated myself to that half-pint of ice cream each week that I stuck to it. I lost over thirty pounds, trimmed over five inches from my waist, and had energy enough to light a major metropolitan area. *It was so painless, so easy*. I looked and felt great. This, from a guy who abhors dieting and exercising. But, like I said, the *Common Sense Approach* didn't *feel* like a diet because I didn't have to give up any type of food, and it didn't force me to exercise. It all just sort of *happened*. And if it happened to me, I just know it can happen for you as well.

I discovered that *anything* can happen if you set your mind to it, and have faith in your beliefs. I honestly believed that I could change my lifestyle if only a program didn't force me to do it all so quickly. When, in my research, I could not find a diet plan that suited me personally, I created one. Not knowing for sure if it would be a success.

I mustered up all the faith I could and was determined to make it work. And it did. I looked at the *Common Sense Approach to a Healthy Lifestyle* as a sort of St. Jude of weight loss -- this was to be the last hope, the last attempt that I would ever make at trying to lose weight.

The *Common Sense Approach* was stylized to accommodate all my little weaknesses, and to play to the few strengths I had. It was customized to require little effort on my part and it encouraged successful focus by its short term approach. In other words, it was a fat man's dream plan. And the great thing was it made perfect sense.

But because it was so sensible and because it was stylized to fit my needs while accomplishing the goals at hand, there was that underlying knowledge that if the *Common Sense Approach to a Healthy Lifestyle* failed, I would remain a Person of Preposterous Proportions for the rest of my life. And, quite frankly, that thought scared the hell out of me. But, at the same time, it enhanced my determination.

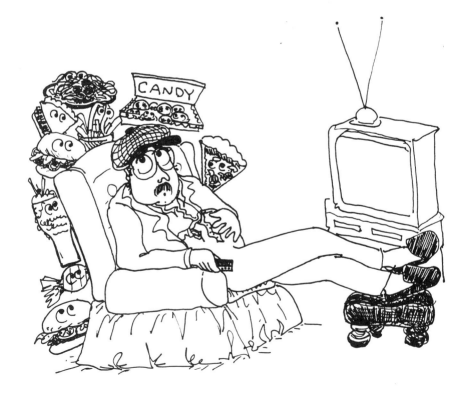

CHAPTER SIX
The Insidious Invasion

I had met the enemy and it was mine. How wonderful it was living the life of a thin person! At long last I had won the Battle of the Bulge. For over four years I had managed to keep myself trim and fit; happy and energetic. It was both strange and exhilarating.

Remember the children's story about a princess who works up the courage to kiss the frog and transforms it into a handsome prince? That's how I felt three months after being on the *Common Sense Approach*. Like a prince. Okay, maybe not as handsome, but still the transformation was absolutely incredible.

Where once a veritable recluse existed now lived a raving social butterfly. The seldom-chosen fat kid in the neighborhood was now on everyone's social calendar. I was involved. I actually even dated on a regular basis -- though I must confess that I never really understood this ritual very well, but that's another story. And, surprise of surprises, I actually met someone of the fairer sex with whom I fell in lust, and eventually married and started a family. My, wasn't life as a *thin* person grand!

That turned out to be the beginning of a nightmare for me: it was at this alleged blissful point in my life that the Insidious Invasion was launched. I did not have a clue as to what was happening.

One day as I got up from my easy chair, I realized that I could no longer see my feet for the size of my stomach.

Oh, God, I thought, *I had become a Person of Profound Poundage again! How could this have happened? Wasn't it just a short time ago that I had beaten the bulge; that I had dropped an enormous amount of weight? And hadn't I worked hard to keep it off? How could I let myself go to hell like this?* I was shocked and appalled as I gaped at my reflection in the mirror. There had been a sneak attack of fat, and it had taken me completely by surprise. And now it held me hostage.

*****

I made a valuable discovery that day. I realized that being prone to weight gain is not unlike being an alcoholic: the venue is different of course, but we share a common state of mind. Just as the recovering alcoholic must guard against the temptation to drink alcohol, so, too, must people who love to eat -- like me -- protect against the appetite. Otherwise, one average serving of food becomes a *generous* portion that soon becomes two ... then three ... and pretty soon, the bulge has returned to the midriff, the clothes are too damned tight, and you're standing in front of a full-length mirror, gaping at a God-awful reflection that makes you want to hurl, scratching your balding head, and wondering: how *did* this happen?

I discovered that complacency is, without doubt, a greater adversary than was the ritual of overeating. It is the greatest enemy that we appetite-challenged people, and others like us, will ever face. Sure there are support groups out there that you can join and lean on, but you must be *aware* that the problem exists -- and ready to *admit* it -- before you can become a groupie. Besides, it seems to me that a better way to solve the situation is to meet it squarely face-to-face. You know, look it right in the eye, give it your best Clint Eastwood-snarl, and then make-its-day type of approach.

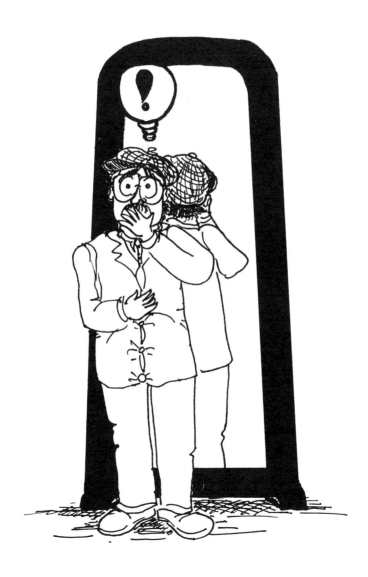

Besides that, doing something yourself -- especially when it is an extremely challenging task -- does wonders in building self-esteem, right? As long as you *succeed*, that is. Well then, doing it yourself does save alot of money!

That's how I solved the situation which confronted me in the mirror that day. After I got done hurling from the sight of my reflection, I got downright angry at myself for being so complacent that I could give in to the Demon Desires of those wonderful foods I loved to eat. I was mad -- *fighting* mad -- at myself. Mad that I'd reverted to that lazy lump of humanity of yesteryear. Mad that I hadn't seen it coming.

I really chewed myself out, but good, over the whole mess. And then I set out to assess the damage. What I learned was shocking. I had jumped in weight to nearly two hundred and forty pounds, and my waist measured forty-five inches! I was actually heavier at that juncture than at any other stage of my life. All because I just plain didn't care enough to keep on top of things.

So what did I do to make amends? I began by analyzing *what* and *when* I ate for an entire week. I visited a physician and went through a physical examination to confirm my suspicions. Does this sound vaguely familiar? Of course it does.

I set out on another campaign to beat the Battle of the Bulge armed with the nuclear bomb of weight loss programs -- the *Common Sense Approach*. I was absolute in my determination to whip my adversary. I hated myself for what I had become and, knowing that I beat it before, somehow made the task ahead a little easier to comprehend.

*****

I developed a new Personal Agenda, followed the Attack Plans, and leaped into the lurch with blind ambition and the desire to show no mercy at the hands of my foe. Trouble was, the second time around was not any easier. In fact, it seemed that the first few days were substantially more demanding than ever before. Around every corner, tucked away in the dark recesses of every cabinet and cupboard, lurked the vile temptation of my foe. I struggled with the bombardment of foodstuffs being lavished upon me. The twilight assaults and sniper attacks were constant and unrelenting in their force.

Near the middle of that first week back on the *Approach*, the pounding inside my stomach escalated to the force of a jackhammer on concrete. I was shellshocked and weary from the constant battles and honestly, I really felt discouraged. My psyche, already fragile from this quirk of Fate that left me fatter than ever, was taking a beating. All those old taunts and jeers, the snide little asides being softly spoken, about my weight gain were murdering me. I wanted to give up and say to hell with it. But then, there was a light. A *vision* ...

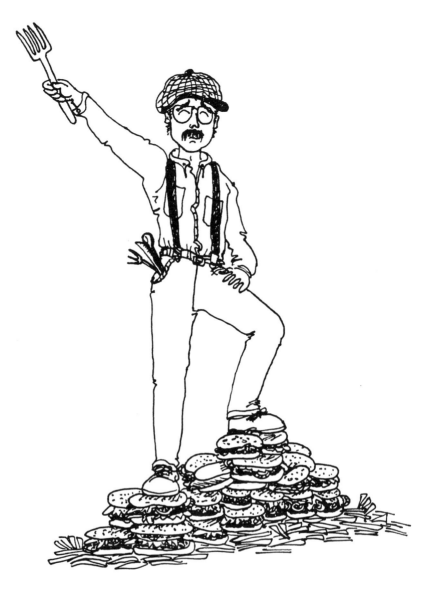

CHAPTER SEVEN
Armistice Day

The light was the one that comes on when you open the refrigerator door. What made it so bright, I suppose, was that I had wandered there under cover of night and with no other lights on, those things shine pretty brightly.

You see, I had decided a few minutes earlier while tossing and turning in bed with visions of sugarplums, among other stuff, dancing in my head, that I was going to quit the *Common Sense Approach* altogether. I was obviously destined to be fat. And, quite frankly, I didn't care at that point as long as I could eat the leftover strawberry shortcake that was beckoning to me from the back of the refrigerator. *Que sera, sera.*

But as I leaned into the confines of the old ice box and reached for my just desserts, something really kind of spooky happened. This image appeared. In my head. For a moment there, I thought I was having one of those really weird religious experiences you often read about, but on closer examination, I realized what it *really* was: my pot o' gold at the end of the rainbow. I saw myself sitting on the steps of the local ice cream parlor eating a half-pint of ice cream. The sun was shining brightly and there I was smiling and looking quite content. And *thin.*

The whole image lasted all of maybe three or four seconds, certainly not any longer than that. But it was just enough for me to close the door and go back upstairs to bed. I knew at that very moment that I had beat the Battle of the Bulge. Again. And as I climbed those stairs that evening, I made a commitment to never again become complacent with regard to my eating and my lifestyle. I acknowledged that I was a Person Prone to Porcine Proportions and would have to live with that for the rest of my life. I accepted it. Plain and simple. And unconditionally.

*****

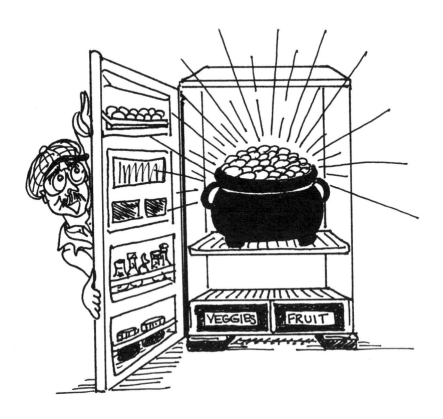

I practiced good old common sense and began modifying my eating habits as diagrammed in the *Common Sense Approach*. Over the next eight months of following the *Approach* I was to lose over seventy-five pounds, and eleven inches from my waist! I had actually **won the war**. Not once, but *twice* ...

That last victory was well over a decade ago. Today, I still practice the *Common Sense Approach* because *it's a way of life*. It's second nature. Certainly, I continue to keep my guard up against the glancing blows of complacency, but I don't *consciously* do it. I've been following the *Approach* for so many years now that I know when to say enough is enough. I have **willpower**. Heck, I've even treated myself to ice cream during the week on a number of occasions without backsliding into those nasty habits.

I've tested the *Approach*. I've pushed it to its limits. And, I'm pleased to say, it has endured. And so have I.

How well have I endured? As this book goes to press, my weight fluctuates between one hundred seventy-four and one hundred seventy-eight pounds; my waist size is thirty-four inches. And I've been eating whatever whenever without guilt or worry. There has been **absolutely no sacrifice**.

No longer do I sit in front of the television feeding my face as my main source of exercise. Now days, I am active in a variety of recreational endeavors like softball and volleyball. I walk or ride a bicycle when it would be far more convenient to hop in my car and drive. Why? Quite simply, **the *Common Sense Approach* revitalized me**. It gave me energy. To burn. And I just plain *feel* good.

Okay, there's nothing else to tell and only one thing left for you to do: get with it. I mentioned this early on, but it merits repeating. I obviously cannot guarantee that the *Common Sense Approach to a Healthy Lifestyle* will work for you. All I can say is that it has worked for me -- not once, but *twice* -- when no other weight reduction plan did.

The *Approach* worked because it was designed specifically with the anti-diet, anti-exercise freak in mind. Me. There are no tricks, no gimmicks, and absolutely no sacrifices. The *Common Sense Approach* is nothing more than good old common sense. That's it.

While guarantees cannot be made, as you read through this book remember that there's a good chance that we share many of the same qualities. I had tried many diet programs, both the conventional and the unorthodox. I spent beaucoups bucks trying to get rid of my ever-expanding waistline without success. Why? Because every diet I ever tried wanted me to work hard at losing weight, and honestly, I just didn't want to. And besides, I was essentially lazy and didn't have an abundance of willpower.

What I discovered was, I do have an abundance of good old common sense. And by capitalizing on that strength I managed to overcome a lot of glaring weaknesses. Like eating too much and exercising all too infrequently. The *Approach* worked for me, and I really believe it will work for you. All you have to do is start -- that's the greatest obstacle and most difficult part of the *Common Sense Approach to a Healthy Lifestyle*. So, get with it!

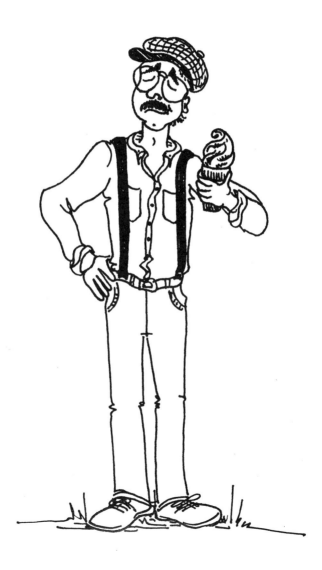

COMMON SENSE APPROACH

If you found the *Common Sense Approach to a Healthy Lifestyle* a useful resource in your efforts to lose weight, please write to us, in care of the publisher, to let us know how you feel about the program. And, don't hesitate to examine the other COMMON SENSE offerings listed below.

ORDER FORM

Name _____

Address _____

City/State _____

Please send me the *Common Sense Books* checked below:

☐ *Common Sense Approach to a Healthy Lifestyle*   #_____
☐ *Common Sense Approach to Getting What You
    Want Out of Life*   #_____
☐ *Common Sense Approach to Parenting One or a
    Whole Bunch of Kids*   #_____

Common Sense Books are $15.95 each, plus $3.00 shipping costs. Make checks payable to **Common Sense Books**.

Please enter my subscription to **Common Sense Primer** newsletter, published quarterly. I have enclosed an additional $25.00 for my annual subscription fee.

Total Number of Books Ordered	@ $15.95 each	_____
Number of *Common Sense Primer*	@ $25.00	_____
Plus Shipping Costs	@ $3.00	_____
Total Amount Enclosed	$ _____	

Please allow 8-10 weeks for delivery of all books and materials ordered.